Guidelines to handling prostate cancer: Understanding prostate Cancer and being the Conqueror

TABLE OF CONTENT

CHAPTER I

Everything about Prostate cancer

What Is the Prostate?

The prostate is a portion of the male reproductive system, which comprises the penis, prostate, seminal vesicles, and testicles. The prostate is placed directly below the bladder and in front of the rectum. It is roughly the size of a walnut and surrounds the urethra (the tube that drains pee from the bladder) (the tube that empties urine from the bladder). It generates fluid that makes up a portion of semen.

As a man matures, the prostate tends to expand in size. This might cause the urethra to constrict and limit urine flow. This is termed benign prostatic hyperplasia, and it is not the same as prostate cancer.

Understanding Prostate Changes

The prostate is a tiny gland in males. It is part of the male reproductive system. The prostate is roughly the size and shape of a walnut. It rests deep in the pelvis, below the bladder and immediately in front of the rectum. The prostate helps create semen, the milky fluid that transfers sperm from the testicles via the penis when a man ejaculates. The prostate surrounds part of the urethra, a tube that transports urine out of the bladder and via the penis.

How the Prostate Changes As You Age

Since the prostate gland tends to become bigger with age, it may constrict the urethra and create difficulty in passing pee. Occasionally men in their 30s and 40s may begin to develop these urine symptoms and require medical intervention. For others, symptoms aren't seen until much later in life. An infection or a tumor may also make the prostate bigger. Be careful to notify your doctor if you develop any of the urinary symptoms mentioned below.

Inform your doctor if you develop these urine symptoms:

- ☐ Are passing pee more throughout the day \sHave an urgent desire to pass urine
- ☐ Have decreased urine flow
- ☐ Felt burning as you pass urine

- [ ] Need to wake up multiple times throughout the night to pass urine
- [ ] Getting older enhances your chance of prostate issues. The three most frequent prostate disorders are inflammation (prostatitis), enlarged prostate (BPH, or benign prostatic hyperplasia), and prostate cancer.

One change does not lead to another. For example, having prostatitis or an enlarged prostate does not enhance your risk of prostate cancer. It is also conceivable for you to have more than one ailment at the same time.

What is prostrate Cancer?

Cancer of the prostate is the second most common cancerous tumor worldwide and is the fifth leading cause of cancer-related mortality among men. The prostate is a gland in the male reproductive system that surrounds the urethra just below the bladder. It is located in the hypogastric region of the abdomen. To give an idea of where it is located, the bladder is superior to the prostate gland as shown in the image The rectum is posterior in perspective to the prostate gland and the ischial tuberosity of the pelvic bone is inferior. Most prostate cancers are slow growing. Cancerous cells may spread to other areas of the body, particularly the bones and lymph nodes. It may initially cause no symptoms. In later stages, symptoms include pain or difficulty urinating, blood in the urine, or pain in the pelvis or back. Benign prostatic hyperplasia may produce similar symptoms. Other late symptoms include fatigue, due to low levels of red blood cells.

Factors that increase the risk of prostate cancer include older age, family history, and race.

About 99% of cases occur after age 50. A first-degree relative with the disease increases the risk two- to three-fold. Additional concerns include a diet heavy on processed meat and red meat, whereas the danger from the high consumption of milk products is uncertain. A correlation with gonorrhea has been established, however, no rationale for this interaction has been identified. A higher risk is connected with BRCA mutations. Diagnosis is by biopsy. Medical imaging may be done to determine if metastasis is present.

Prostate cancer screening, including prostate-specific antigen (PSA) testing, enhances cancer diagnosis but whether it improves outcomes is debatable. Informed decision-making is advised for adults 55 to 69 years old. Testing, if carried out, is more suitable for persons with a longer life expectancy. While 5α-reductase inhibitors seem to lower low-grade cancer risk, they do not impact high-grade cancer risk, therefore are not advised for prevention. Vitamin or mineral supplementation does not seem to impact risk.

Many instances are handled with active observation or careful waiting. Additional treatments may involve a combination of surgery, radiation therapy, hormone therapy, or chemotherapy. Tumors localized to the prostate may be treatable. Pain medicines, bisphosphonates, and targeted therapy,[21] among others, may be beneficial. Results depend on age, health state, and how aggressive and widespread the cancer is. [2] Most men with prostate cancer do not die from it. The United States' five-year survival rate is 98%.

Worldwide, it is the second-most frequent cancer. It is the fifth-leading cause of cancer-related mortality among males. In 2018, it was diagnosed in 1.2 million and caused 359,000 fatalities. It was the most prevalent cancer among men in 84 nations, appearing more often in the industrialized world. Rates have been growing in the emerging world. Detection grew considerably in the 1980s and 1990s in several locations owing to increasing PSA testing. One research revealed prostate cancer in 30% to 70% of Russian and Japanese men over age 60 who had died of unrelated causes.

The reality of prostrate cancer for males

Prostate cancer affects predominantly elderly males. Six out of ten instances are diagnosed in males over 65, but fewer than 1% in men under 50. While rare, prostate cancer may be observed in males even in their 30s and 40s. Males with a family history of prostate cancer are more likely to get prostate cancer than the general population.

On a case-by-case basis, physicians cannot declare with precision what causes prostate cancer, although experts generally agree that nutrition adds to the risk. Men who consume big quantities of fat — notably from red meat and other forms of animal fat cooked at high heat — may be more prone to develop advanced prostate cancer. The condition is significantly more frequent in nations where meat and dairy products are dietary mainstays than in countries where the fundamental diet consists of rice, soybean products, and vegetables such as broccoli, cauliflower, cole slaw, or sauerkraut.

The fundamental factor connecting food and prostate cancer is probably hormonal. Fats induce increased production of testosterone and other hormones, and testosterone serves to expedite the formation of prostate cancer. High testosterone levels may drive latent prostate cancer cells into action. Several data imply that elevated testosterone levels can impact the earliest start of prostate cancer.

Welders, battery producers, rubber workers, and workers often exposed to the chemical cadmium tend to be unusually prone to prostate cancer.

The following are also connected with an increased risk of advanced prostate cancer: Height, high body mass index, poor physical activity, smoking, low tomato sauce consumption, high calcium intake, high linoleic acid intake, African-American race, and positive family history.

No documented relationship exists between prostate cancer with an active sex life, vasectomy, masturbation, use of alcohol or cigarettes, circumcision, infertility, infection of the prostate, or a common noncancerous disease termed benign prostatic hyperplasia (BPH) (BPH). Most, if not all, men will suffer an enlarged prostate as they age.

CHAPTER II

Prostate Cancer in Black Males

African men are half as likely to die of prostate cancer now as they were a few decades ago. That's excellent news. Yet, there remain racial differences when it comes to early diagnosis, treatment, and fatalities.

Speak to your doctor about your risk. Researchers urge Black men to discuss that and prepare for future testing by age 45. Here's more on how prostate cancer affects Black males.

How Does Prostate Cancer Impact, Black Men?

Prostate cancer accounts for 37% of all malignancies in Black males. Roughly 1 in 6 will be diagnosed with the condition at some point in life. It's more frequent among Black guys than other racial/ethnic groupings.

The illness is especially deadlier for African guys. They're twice as likely to die from prostate cancer compared to guys of other races. That's the highest racial differential in fatalities from any malignancy in the United States.

When it comes to prostate cancer, Black men are also more susceptible than other races to:

- Be diagnosed at an early age
- Have fast-growing, or high-grade, tumor cells
- Having prostate cancer that has spread to other regions of the body (called advanced or metastatic cancer) (called advanced or metastatic cancer)
- We have a greater knowledge of prostate cancer in Black males than we used to, but more study is required. Racial minorities are routinely excluded from clinical research for numerous reasons. Yet there's a rising movement to include more Black males in research studies.

Why Does Prostate Cancer Affect Black Men Differently?

Health inequalities are mostly blamed on decades of racial prejudice and discrimination. You may hear this dubbed systemic or structural racism. It may affect every element of life, including access to nutritious food, work, housing, and medical treatment.

Yet researchers are still striving to uncover explanations for precisely why prostate cancer is more frequent and lethal in Black men. Such hypotheses include:

Barriers to care. Black males frequently have poorer access to health insurance and high-quality medical treatment. Access to medical care, education, work, and money all affect how healthy you are. If you're a Black guy with prostate cancer, racial and socioeconomic hurdles may contribute to:

- Delays in therapy
- Reduced rates of prostate cancer screenings
- Little health education regarding treatment options
- Poor quality care
- Fewer high-benefit procedures, such as surgery
- Terrible advice. From 2012 to 2018, the U.S. Preventative Services Task Force (USPSTF)

declared they didn't believe the PSA test should be used for regular prostate cancer screening. That's a blood test routinely used to identify early symptoms of prostate cancer. They've altered their recommendations since then, stating that men should make that choice with their physicians depending on their risk of prostate cancer. Yet other experts say the advice against PSA screening likely inflicted a harsher toll on Black males compared to other races.

Medical distrust. Black folks are frequently less trusting of the healthcare system. There are cultural and historical reasons behind this.

Fewer Black physicians. Individuals may feel more comfortable with a doctor who shares their race. Although 13% of the population is Black, just 5% of the employment comprises Black physicians. And barely 2% of urologists are Black. Urologists are professionals who commonly diagnose and treat prostate cancer.

Additional health difficulties. Your lifestyle, such as what you eat and whether you exercise or smoke, coupled with your genes, influences your health. And the constant stress of systematic racism may also make you ill.

Some medical disorders occur more commonly in Black males. Factors that might adversely influence prostate cancer outcomes include:

- Heart disease
- Diabetes
- Overweight or obesity
- Genetic variations. Genes are handed down via families. And there's some indication that Black males may inherit the risk for more aggressive kinds of cancer or specific genetic abnormalities, or alterations.

There's a continuous dispute regarding how much biology affects prostate cancer in Black men. We may know more in the future if genetic testing becomes generally accessible.

CHAPTER III

Risk Factors of prostate cancer

A risk factor is something that enhances a person's likelihood of acquiring cancer. While risk factors typically impact the potential to acquire cancer, most do not directly or by themselves cause cancer. Some persons with numerous recognized risk factors never acquire cancer, whereas others with no known risk factors do. Understanding your risk factors and talking about them with your doctor may help you make better-educated lifestyle and healthcare decisions.

The following variables may boost a person's chance of acquiring prostate cancer:

Age. The risk of prostate cancer rises with age, particularly after age 50. Roughly 60% of prostate malignancies are detected in patients who are 65 or older. Older persons who are diagnosed with prostate cancer might encounter significant problems, notably concerning cancer treatment. For further information, please read Cancer.Net's section regarding aging and cancer.

Race. Black males in the United States, and other men of African descent, are diagnosed with prostate cancer more than men of other races. Black men are more likely to die from prostate cancer than White men.

North American or northern European place. Prostate cancer occurs more commonly in North America and northern Europe. It also suggests that prostate cancer is growing among Asian individuals living in urbanized surroundings, such as Hong Kong, Singapore, North American, and European cities, especially among those who lead a lifestyle with less physical activity and a less nutritious diet.

Family history. Prostate cancer that runs in a family, termed familial prostate cancer, accounts for 20% of all prostate cancers. This form of prostate cancer occurs due to a combination of common genes and shared environmental or lifestyle factors.

Hereditary prostate cancer, inheriting the risk from a relative, is uncommon and accounts for roughly 5%

of all occurrences. Hereditary prostate cancer arises when variations in genes, or mutations, are handed down within a family from 1 generation to the next. This is termed a germline mutation. If someone has a first-degree relative—meaning a parent, sibling, or child—with prostate cancer, their chance of acquiring prostate cancer is 2 to 3 times greater than the usual risk. This risk rises even higher with the number of relatives diagnosed with prostate cancer.

Hereditary prostate cancer may be suspected if a family history contains any of the following characteristics:

3 or more first-degree relatives with prostate cancer

Prostate cancer in 3 generations on the same side of the family, 2 or more close relatives, such as a parent, sibling, child, grandparent, uncle, or nephew, on the same side of the family, diagnosed with prostate cancer before age 55.

Hereditary breast and ovarian cancer (HBOC) syndrome. HBOC is related to the germline, or inherited, DNA-repair mutations to the BRCA1 and/or BRCA2 genes. BRCA stands for "BReast

CAncer." HBOC is most typically related to an elevated risk of breast and ovarian malignancies in women. Nevertheless, men with HBOC also have an increased chance of acquiring breast cancer and a more severe type of prostate cancer. Mutations in the BRCA1 and BRCA2 genes are thought to cause only a small percentage of inherited prostate cancers. Individuals who have BRCA1 or BRCA2 mutations should consider screening for prostate cancer at an earlier age. Genetic testing may only be useful for families with prostate cancer that may also have HBOC. If you are concerned about this based on your family history, please talk with a genetic counselor or doctor for more information.

Other genetic changes. Other genes that may carry an increased risk of developing prostate cancer include HPC1, HPC2, HPCX, CAPB, ATM, FANCA, HOXB13, and mismatch repair genes. However, none of them has been directly shown to cause prostate cancer or be specific to this disease. Research to identify genes associated with an increased risk of prostate cancer is ongoing, and researchers are constantly learning more about how specific genetic changes can influence the development of prostate cancer. At present, there are no genetic tests available to determine someone's chance of developing prostate cancer.

Agent Orange exposure. The U.S. Department of Veterans Affairs (VA) lists prostate cancer as a disease associated with exposure to Agent Orange, a chemical used during the Vietnam War. If you are a veteran who may have been exposed to Agent Orange, please speak to your doctor in the VA system. Read more about the relationship with Agent Orange in this article.

Eating habits and weight. No research has demonstrated that food and nutrition may directly cause or prevent the development of prostate cancer. Yet, much research that looks at relationships between various eating practices and cancer shows there may be a connection. For example, obesity is connected with many malignancies, including prostate cancer, and a balanced diet to minimize weight gain is suggested (see "Dietary changes" below).

The substantial facts concerning prostrate cancer that guys should take heed of

Prostate cancer is often a slow-growing kind of cancer that has a likelihood of excellent survival when identified early. That's why it's crucial to understand more about it, including some of the most unexpected facts concerning this form of cancer. The more you know, the more likely you'll be to notice when anything is odd and get checked out by your doctor.

Here, I have put together a list of some of the lesser-known facts concerning prostate cancer.

1. Most Men Survive Prostate Cancer

Although a prostate cancer diagnosis might come with many emotions, the good news is that the survival rate is excellent. Ninety-five percent of all prostate cancer cases are discovered when the malignancy is still within the prostate. While cancer is still restricted to one region, it makes it much simpler to discover and treat.

Additionally, 99% of men diagnosed with prostate cancer survive at least five years following the diagnosis. Although these figures are hopeful, it's still vital to enhance your chances of survival by consulting with your doctor and scheduling any prescribed prostate cancer exams. Early diagnosis is crucial and may have a huge influence on your treatment choices.

2. Prostate Cancer May Affect Younger Men Too

Although the average age of prostate cancer diagnosis is indeed 66 years old, younger men might still be diagnosed. The reality is, that prostate cancer in younger men (below the age of 50) is frequently more aggressive and may spread quicker, which makes it more difficult to cure. Because of this, men aged 40 and above should be particularly watchful of any changes in their health. Some signs of prostate cancer to be aware of include:

- Frequent urination
- Blood in your pee
- Weak urine flow

The unexpected desire to pee in the middle of the night \sPain or burning while urinating
Screening recommendations from the American Cancer Society include:

Age 50 for males who have an average risk of prostate cancer

Age 45 for males with a high risk of prostate cancer. High-risk factors include having an immediate family member under the age of 65 who has been diagnosed with prostate cancer or if you are an African American.

3. Prostate Cancer Symptoms Mimic Other Diseases

The symptoms stated above signal that there are malignant cells inside the prostate, however, the symptoms are comparable to various other illnesses or ailments of the prostate or urinary system. They might sometimes be so subtle that they go undetected for a long.

Some men don't have any symptoms, particularly if it is identified early. However, men who suffer any of these symptoms should speak to their doctor. In many circumstances, they will undertake a physical check and offer a prostate cancer screening test, particularly if they are 50 or older. It's always advisable to arrange an appointment with your doctor sooner rather than later if you see anything strange.

4. There May be a Genetic Connection to Prostate Cancer

Age and lifestyle may contribute to the development of prostate cancer. Yet, research reveals that inherited factors may be a cause. A BRCA1 or BRCA2 gene mutation has been confirmed to lead to prostate cancer (the same gene mutation connected with certain breast cancers) (the same gene mutation associated with breast cancers). Read more about the gene panel testing that may discover cancer-associated mutations. Those who have other men in their families who have been diagnosed with prostate cancer should check themselves constantly and visit their physician to search for the indicators of prostate cancer.

Researchers are not convinced of the precise relationship between the BRCA gene and this form of cancer. Nonetheless, they have observed that males with this gene mutation increase the chance of a prostate cancer diagnosis.

5. Prostate Cancer is More Frequent Than You Thought

Alongside skin cancer, prostate cancer is the most often diagnosed cancer among males in the US. 1 in 9 American males will be diagnosed with prostate cancer at some point in their lives.

6. Cancer Therapy May Not Always Be The First Option

Most individuals think that cancer always demands quick treatment. Unfortunately, this isn't always the case for prostate cancer individuals with the slow-growing kind of disease.

Occasionally there are signals of prostate cancer in laboratory testing, but few symptoms emerge elsewhere. An oncologist may propose that waiting and monitoring the patient is the best strategy ahead in certain circumstances. This is termed cautious waiting. Don't miss the appointments for subsequent testing to assess if cancer looks to be developing.

Individuals who are advanced in age may not be the greatest candidates for early therapy. Some prostate cancer therapies, such as radiation or chemotherapy, may exert a tremendous amount of stress on the body and worsen general health in older people. In certain circumstances, your doctor may just elect to test occasionally to monitor cancer's progress. In the interim, you should also check for further symptoms and let your doctor know so therapy modifications may be made.

7. Prostate Cancer is More Frequent among Black American Males

Study reveals that African American males are 60% more likely to acquire prostate cancer than white men. Yet, a prostate cancer diagnosis is less prevalent in Hispanic or Asian males. African American men should be especially diligent about prostate cancer screenings due to the higher risk.

8. Lifestyle May Affect Risk of Developing Prostate Cancer

A sedentary (inactive) lifestyle can increase the chance of developing cancerous prostate cells. Diet can also play a role in the likeliness of developing various types of cancer. Research indicates that eating a healthy, balanced diet may decrease your risk of various conditions, including prostate cancer.

Common Misconceptions about Prostate Cancer

• Prostate cancer is an old man's disease.

• If you don't…show more content…
• Stage II cancer involves more than one part of the prostate.

• Stage III cancer has spread beyond the outer layer of the prostate into nearby tissue.

• Stage IV cancer has progressed to other regions of the body such as the bladder, bone, liver, and lungs.

CHAPTER IV

How to treat prostate Cancer

Various methods of therapy are available for prostate cancer. You and your doctor will determine which therapy is suitable for you. Some typical therapies are—

Expectant management. If your doctor feels your prostate cancer is unlikely to develop fast, he or she may suggest that you don't treat the disease right immediately. Alternatively, you might opt to wait and see whether you acquire symptoms in one of two ways:

Active surveillance. Carefully monitoring prostate cancer by doing prostate-specific antigen (PSA) testing and prostate biopsies periodically, and treating cancer only if it develops or produces symptoms.

Watchful waiting. No tests are done. Your doctor addresses any symptoms as they emerge. This is normally indicated for males who are projected to survive for 10 more years or fewer.

Surgery. A prostatectomy is a procedure in which physicians remove the prostate. Radical prostatectomy eliminates the prostate as well as the surrounding tissue.

Radiation treatment. Utilizing high-energy radiation (similar to X-rays) to eliminate cancer. There are two forms of radiation therapy—

External radiation treatment. Equipment outside the body directs radiation to the cancer cells.

Internal radiation treatment (brachytherapy) (brachytherapy). Radioactive seeds or pellets are surgically implanted into or around the malignancy to eliminate the cancer cells.

Additional medicines utilized in the treatment of prostate cancer that is currently under development include—

Cryotherapy. Putting a specific probe within or near the prostate cancer to freeze and destroy the cancer cells.

Chemotherapy. Employing specific medications to shrink or destroy cancer. The medications might be tablets you swallow or medicines administered via your veins, or, occasionally, both.

Biological treatment. Works with your body's immune system to help it fight cancer or to reduce adverse effects from other cancer therapies. Side effects are how your body responds to medications or other therapies.

High-intensity focused ultrasound. This treatment delivers high-energy sound waves (ultrasound) toward the malignancy to eliminate cancer cells.
Hormone treatment. Prevent cancer cells from acquiring the hormones they need to flourish.

Complementary and Alternative Medicine

Complementary and alternative medicines are medications and health practices that are not traditional cancer therapies. Complementary medicine is used in addition to regular therapies, while alternative medicine is used instead of traditional treatments. Meditation, yoga, and supplements like vitamins and herbs are among examples.

Several forms of complementary and alternative medicine have not been tested scientifically and may not be safe. Speak to your doctor about the dangers and benefits before you start any sort of supplementary or alternative medication.
Immunotherapy for Prostate Cancer.

Immunotherapy is a method of cancer treatment. It employs compounds created by the body or in a laboratory to stimulate the immune system and assist the body to detect and kill cancer cells.

Immunotherapy can treat many different forms of cancer. It may be used alone or in conjunction with chemotherapy and/or other cancer therapies.

The immune system comprises a complicated mechanism that your body utilizes to combat cancer. This process includes cells, organs, and proteins. Cancer may often get beyond many of the immune system's natural defenses, enabling cancer cells to continue to thrive.

Various forms of immunotherapy function in different ways. Certain immunotherapy therapies assist the immune system block or limiting the development of cancer cells. Others assist the immune system attack cancer cells or blocking cancer from spreading to other regions of the body.

The many kinds of immunotherapy include:

Monoclonal antibodies and immune checkpoint inhibitors

Non-specific immunotherapies

Oncolytic virus treatment

T-cell therapy

Cancer vaccinations

The kind of immunotherapy, dosage and treatment plan your doctor advises will depend on numerous variables. These can include the type of cancer, size, location, and where it has spread. Your age, general health, body weight, and possible side effects are also important. Talk with your doctor about why a specific immunotherapy plan is being recommended for you.

Surgery and radiation treat prostate cancer by removing or killing cancer cells. Immunotherapy is different. It trains your immune system to attack cancer.

Cancer vaccines and checkpoint inhibitors are approved immunotherapies for prostate cancer. CAR T-cell therapy is a new treatment that doctors are learning more about in clinical trials

You could be a good candidate for one of these therapies if your cancer didn't stop growing or it came back after surgery or hormone therapy. Immunotherapy might help some individuals with prostate cancer survive longer, but it does have certain dangers to discuss with your doctor.

Prostate Cancer Vaccine – Sipuleucel-T (Provenge) (Provenge)

Most immunizations protect you from becoming ill. They prepare your immune system to spot pathogens and fight against them. Sipuleucel-T is a distinct sort of vaccination. It heals cancer by instructing your immune system to detect and destroy cancer cells.

Sipuleucel-T can't treat everyone who has prostate cancer. It could be a possibility for you if:

Your prostate cancer has spread.
You have minimal or no symptoms.
Hormone treatment for your prostate cancer hasn't helped. Such therapy utilizes medications or surgery to suppress the hormones your cancer requires to develop.

Sipuleucel-T is the only authorized prostate cancer vaccination. It's tailor-made for you using your immune cells.

To give you this therapy, initially, your medical team links you to a machine that filters some of the immune cells out of your blood. You go back home. The sample of cells travels to a lab. The lab staff exposes them to a protein that activates the cells and trains them to fight prostate cancer.

After the cells are ready around 3 days later, you visit your doctor's office or hospital again. They deliver the powered-up cells back to you through an IV. You get three doses in total, 2 weeks apart. Each dose takes about an hour.

Sipuleucel-T doesn't stop prostate cancer cells from proliferating. It also doesn't reduce your level of PSA, a protein in your blood that suggests prostate cancer. Yet it could help you live longer.

If you suffer adverse effects with sipuleucel-T, they generally start after you obtain the IV of the treated cells. The most prevalent adverse effects of sipuleucel-T are like the flu:

Chills \sTiredness
Fever

Back and joint pain

Nausea \sHeadache

They should fade away in 1 to 2 days and are generally mild to severe. A tiny minority of patients suffer more serious symptoms such as problems breathing and high blood pressure. Your medical team can address these symptoms.

Checkpoint Inhibitors

Checkpoints are proteins that help prostate cancer hide from your immune system. Checkpoint inhibitors disrupt these proteins to increase your immune response to cancer. These may help reduce PSA levels in those who have previously tried other prostate cancer therapies.

Pembrolizumab (Keytruda) and dostarlimab (Jemperli) are checkpoint inhibitors. They inhibit a protein called PD-1 in immune cells. Blocking PD-1 is like taking the breaks off immune cells so they can fight prostate cancer. You receive this therapy via an IV roughly once every 3 weeks.

These medicines only work for persons who have particular mutations to genes that mend damaged DNA. Up to 10% of men with late-stage prostate cancer had these gene alterations, which often afflict patients with a hereditary disorder called Lynch syndrome.

Your medical team will test for these gene alterations in a piece of your cancer that they remove during a biopsy. The test may reveal if a checkpoint inhibitor is good for you.

If you do suffer adverse effects with a checkpoint inhibitor, they could feel like the flu. Some of the most frequent symptoms include weariness, coughing, nausea, diarrhea, and appetite loss.

Checkpoint inhibitors fire up your immune system so they can attack your cancer. Occasionally, the immune system revs up too much and targets healthy organs like the lungs, kidneys, or liver. If that occurs, your care team could

CAR T-Cell Therapy

T cells are your immune system's army of cancer fighters. CAR T-cell therapy is an investigational treatment that teaches your T cells to locate and destroy prostate cancer. At now, you can only acquire this medicine in a clinical study.

To obtain CAR T-cell treatment, initially, your medical team will link you to a machine that filters

T cells out of your blood. In a lab, the team places a protein called a chimeric antigen receptor on the exterior of your cells. This protein will assist your T cells to detect malignancy.

The lab generates many more of the new CAR T cells, which may take a few weeks. After the cells are ready, you go back to your doctor's office and obtain them via an IV.

This therapy might induce adverse effects. When CAR T cells grow, your body produces substances called cytokines. A surge of cytokines might fire up the immune system too much. The nomenclature for this adverse effect is cytokine release syndrome (CRS) (CRS). It produces symptoms like:

- High fever
- Difficulty breathing
- Nausea, vomiting, and diarrhea
- Dizziness
- Headache
- Rapid heartbeat
-

CAR T-cell treatment may potentially impact the brain. If it does, you can experience symptoms including headaches, disorientation, or seizures. Your medical team will follow you extremely carefully and handle any issues that arise.

CAR T-cell treatment has helped some individuals with blood malignancies go into remission, meaning there were no indications of their malignancy. It hasn't worked as effectively against prostate cancer. One explanation is that solid tumors have additional barriers that hinder T cells from reaching the malignancy. Prostate cancer also inhibits the immune system response.

Doctors are exploring different CAR T-cell therapy to determine whether they perform better against prostate cancer. A CAR T-cell treatment called P-PSMA-101 helped decrease PSA by more than 50% in a few men, and it made one tumor vanish.

CHAPTER V

Prostatectomy: What to Expect During Surgery and Recovery

Prostatectomy Surgery Fundamentals

At Johns Hopkins, surgeons employ the newest methods to conduct prostatectomies. There are two ways surgeons might employ while doing a prostatectomy. With each of these procedures, the final aim is the same - remove the prostate and eliminate cancer.

Robotic surgery: Small incisions and robotic technology allow surgeons to conduct a precise, less invasive treatment with quicker recovery time and fewer incisions.

Open surgery: This method involves typical incisions and instruments. For more difficult conditions, open surgery may be a more suitable alternative than a robotic operation.

A prostatectomy takes roughly two hours. You will be under general anesthesia, so you'll be entirely sleeping. During the procedure, your doctor will:

Create a tiny incision to obtain access to your prostate.

Remove the prostate.
Reconnect the bladder to the urethra, the tube that transports pee outside of the body.
Attach a catheter to the bladder, which permits urine to drain as the region heals.

Following Prostatectomy: What to Expect

In the hospital: You should anticipate being in the hospital for one night. At Johns Hopkins, all rooms on the urology level are private. Here, nurses assist patients to begin moving quickly after surgery to minimize blood clots and other postoperative hazards.

First few days at home: Once you're sent home, you could find that normal ibuprofen or acetaminophen will be adequate pain treatment for the first few days. If over-the-counter drugs aren't adequate, your doctor may assist you with alternatives.

One week following surgery: When your operation site heals, your catheter will be removed. This is commonly seven to 10 days following surgery. This may readily be done in your doctor's office. Some patients elect to take remove their catheter at home. If that's the case, consult your doctor for instructions beforehand.

This is also approximately the time your surgeon will contact you with the final pathology findings. He or she will explain what you should know and if additional therapy is required. (Many guys do not require any additional therapy.)

One month after surgery: Doctors suggest avoiding excessive activities or heavy lifting for at least one month following surgery. Usually, individuals take off work for three to four weeks. If you work from home, you might return to work sooner.

Within one month following surgery, your life should start going back to normal. Some males have adverse effects, including:

Urinary incontinence (urine leakage) (urine leaking)

Erectile dysfunction

Recovering following surgery takes time. These adverse effects are frequently transitory. But, if they are harming your quality of life, ask your doctor about choices that might assist.